Introduction

1/What is losing weight

decreasing body fat is the process of decreasing weight. It can be accomplished by combining dietary modifications, physical activity, and lifestyle adjustments.

People make the decision to reduce weight for a variety of reasons. While some people want to feel and look better, others seek to enhance their health. Losing weight can also help lower the chance of developing chronic illnesses including type 2 diabetes, heart disease, and stroke.

There are several approaches to weight loss. While some people prefer to focus on improving their physical activity, others opt to adhere to a certain diet. There is no one weight reduction strategy that works for everyone; what works for one person might not work for another.

Finding a strategy that you can follow and that makes you feel good is the most crucial step. Speak to your doctor or a certified dietician if you are having trouble losing weight on your own. They can assist you in developing a strategy that is appropriate for you.

<u>Here are a few advantages of losing weight:</u>

- better health
- lower chance of developing chronic disorders
- improved self-esteem and increased vitality
- improved sleep more mobility

Consult with your doctor first if you're thinking about reducing weight. They may advise you on how to lose weight safely and successfully and assist you in determining whether weight reduction is the correct choice for you.

2/ Why is losing weight important

There are several factors that make losing weight crucial. Among the most significant advantages of losing weight are:

- Health improvement: Losing weight can help you feel better overall and lower your chances of developing chronic conditions including heart disease, stroke, type 2 diabetes, and some cancers.
- Reduced risk of chronic diseases: Losing weight can help lower your chance of getting some cancers, heart conditions, strokes, type 2 diabetes, and other chronic illnesses.
- Increased energy levels: Losing weight might help you feel more energized, awake, and attentive.
- Self-esteem: Losing weight might help you feel better about yourself and more confident.
- Better sleep: Losing weight can help you have better quality sleep and find it simpler to go to and remain asleep.
- Mobility improvement: Losing weight can help you move more easily and enhance your mobility.

3/ What are the benefits of weight loss

- Health improvement: Losing weight can help you feel better overall and lower your chances of developing chronic conditions including heart disease, stroke, type 2 diabetes, and some cancers.
- Reduced risk of chronic diseases: Losing weight can help lower your chance of getting some cancers, heart conditions, strokes, type 2 diabetes, and other chronic illnesses.

- Increased energy levels: Losing weight might help you feel more energized, awake, and attentive.
- Self-esteem: Losing weight might help you feel better about yourself and more confident.
- Better sleep: Losing weight can help you have better quality sleep and find it simpler to go to and remain asleep.
- Mobility improvement: Losing weight can help you move more easily and enhance your mobility.
- problems relief: Losing weight might aid in easing joint and other physical problems.
- Weight loss can aid in improving both male and female fertility.
- Reduced risk of heart disease and stroke thanks to decreased blood pressure: Losing weight can help lower blood pressure.
- Reduced risk of heart disease and stroke due to decreased cholesterol: Losing weight can help lower cholesterol levels.
- Better blood sugar regulation: People with type 2 diabetes who lose weight have better blood sugar regulation.

Chapter 1: Setting realistic weight loss goals

1/Introduction

Setting realistic weight loss goals is critical to success. If you set your goals too high, you are more likely to get discouraged and give up. On the other hand, if you set your goals too low, you may not see any progress and get discouraged.

2/SMART target frame

A great way to set realistic weight loss goals is with the SMART goal frame. **SMART** goals are **specific**, **measurable**, **achievable**, **relevant** and **time bound**.

•Clear Goals should be specific and measurable. For example, instead of saying, "I want to lose weight," you can say, "He wants to lose 10 pounds in six months.

•Measurable Goals should be measurable so that progress can be tracked. For example, you can track your weight loss weekly.

•Reachable goals should be achievable but challenging. If the goal is too simple, you will probably not be motivated to achieve it. If your goal is too difficult, you are more likely to give up.

•related Goals should be related to your overall health and fitness goals. For example, if you're trying to improve your cardiovascular health, your weight loss goals should align with that goal

•Expired Goals should have specific deadlines. This will help you stay on track and stay motivated.

3/How to track your process

Record your weight regularly. This is the main way to track your progress. You can weigh yourself daily, weekly, or monthly, depending on your preference.
Track your body measurements. In addition to tracking your weight, you can also track body measurements such as your waist, hips, and chest. This helps you track your fat loss progress.

Track your food intake. If you're serious about losing weight, it's important to monitor your dietary intake. This will help identify areas where you can change your diet. There are many ways to track your food intake, such as using a food diary or calorie counting app. Track your training habits. Tracking your exercise habits is also important. By doing so, you can ensure that you are getting enough exercise and not overdoing it. Track your training habits by logging the types of exercises you do, the duration of your training sessions, and the intensity of your training sessions.

Take progress photos. Taking progress photos is a great way to visually track your progress. This can be especially motivating when you see how far you've come.
Reward yourself for your progress. When you reach your goal, do something fun for yourself and reward yourself. This will help you stay motivated and stay on track. Tracking your weight loss process will help you stay motivated and on track. By following these tips, you can track your progress and see how far you've come.

Here are some additional tips for tracking your weight loss process.

Be consistent. The key to tracking progress is consistency. Monitor your weight, body measurements, food intake, and exercise habits regularly. Be honest. It's important to be honest with yourself when tracking your progress. Do not try to hide anything from yourself or your tracking system.

Be patient. Weight loss takes time and effort. Don't expect to see results overnight. If you keep at it, you will eventually reach your goal.

Tracking your weight loss process is a great way to stay motivated and stay on track. By following these tips, you can track your progress and see how far you've come.

Chapter 2: Making healthy changes to your diet

1/How to eat healthier

Eat lots of fruits and vegetables. Fruits and vegetables are low in calories and rich in nutrients. It's a great way to feel full without overeating.

Choose whole grains over processed grains. Whole grains are a good source of dietary fiber, which helps you feel full and satisfied. Lean protein is essential for weight loss. Protein helps build muscle and burn fat. Choose lean protein sources such as chicken, fish, beans, and lentils.

Limit unhealthy fats. Unhealthy fats, such as saturated and trans fats, can increase your risk of heart disease and other health problems. Limit sugary drinks. Sugary drinks are high in calories and can contribute to weight gain. Drink water, unsweetened tea, or coffee instead. Read food labels carefully. Food labels help you make informed decisions about the foods you eat. Be aware of the calorie, fat, sugar, and sodium content of the food you are considering. Cook more meals at home. When cooking at home, you have more control over the ingredients in your food. This will help you make healthier choices.

Make some changes to your diet. Don't try to change your entire diet overnight. Start with small changes, such as adding more fruits and vegetables to your diet and eating less sugary drinks.

be patient. It takes time to permanently change your eating habits. Don't be discouraged if you don't see immediate results. If you keep at it, you will eventually reach your goal.

A healthier diet is important for losing weight and improving overall health. By following these tips, you can change your diet in a healthy way and reach your weight loss goals.

Here are some additional tips for a healthier diet.

Find healthy recipes that you enjoy. There are many great cookbooks and websites that offer healthy recipes. Find your favorite recipe that fits your lifestyle.

Offer healthy snacks. It's important to have a healthy snack when you're hungry. So avoid unhealthy snacks like potato chips and cookies.

Plan your meals in advance. By planning your meals in advance, you can make healthy choices and avoid unhealthy snacking.

Cook with your family and friends. Cooking with family and friends is a way to enjoy healthier meals. You can share recipes and ideas and support each other on your weight loss journey.

Eating healthier is a journey, not a destination. By following these tips, you can change your diet in a healthy way and reach your weight loss goals.

2/How to read food labels

Beware of portion size. Serving size is the amount of food that counts as one serving. Calories and other nutrients are listed per serving, so it's important to know how many servings are in the package.
Look at the calories A calorie is the amount of energy that food provides. If you want to lose weight, you should use low-calorie foods.
Check fat content. Fat content is the amount of fat in a food. There are many different types of fat, so it's important to know which types of fat are healthy and which are unhealthy.
Consider sugar content. Carbohydrate content is the amount of sugar contained in food. Sugar can contribute to weight gain, so it's important to limit your intake of sugar-containing foods.
Look at the sodium content. Sodium content is the amount of salt in food. Excess sodium intake can raise blood pressure, so it's important to limit your intake of salty foods. Please read the ingredient list. An ingredient list is a list of all ingredients in a food product. This helps identify unhealthy ingredients like trans fats and artificial sweeteners.
Here are some additional tips for reading food labels.

Compare different brands. Different brands of the same food may have different nutritional content. Therefore, it is recommended to compare different brands before deciding on one.
Please pay attention to the portion size. Portion sizes are often smaller than expected. So if you eat it multiple times, you're getting more calories and other nutrients.
Please do not hesitate to ask questions. If you have any questions about what is on the food label, ask a store clerk or registered dietitian.
Reading food labels can help you make informed decisions about the foods you eat. By following these tips, you can be sure of making healthy food choices that work for you.

3/How to make healthy choices at restaurants

Start with a healthy appetizer. Many restaurants offer salads, grilled vegetables, and healthy entrees like hummus and flatbreads. This will help you feel full before your main course and prevent you from overeating.
Choose low-fat proteins. Lean protein is a good source of protein that helps you feel full and satisfied. Choose lean protein sources such as grilled chicken, fish, and tofu.
order vegetables. Vegetables are low in calories and rich in nutrients. It's a great way to increase the size of your meal without adding too many calories.
Ask for sauce and dressing on the side. Sauces and dressings can add a lot of calories and fat to your diet. Ask for it on the side so you can control how much you use.
Share your meal with a friend. If you're trying to lose weight, it's a good idea to share meals with a friend. That way, you can eat less without feeling deficient. Create a healthy alternative. If you don't know what to order, ask the waiter for reasonable alternatives. For example, you can ask for brown rice instead of white rice, or grilled chicken instead of fried chicken.
Please pay attention to the portion size. The portions in restaurants are often much higher than what you eat at home. Please pay attention to the portion size and if you can't eat it all, don't hesitate to ask for a take-out box.
Here are some additional tips for making healthy choices at restaurants.

Be aware of your own triggers. Why are you more likely to order unhealthy food at a restaurant? Once you know your triggers, you can start developing strategies to avoid them.
Please plan ahead. If you know you'll be eating out, plan ahead and choose a restaurant with a healthy menu. You can even browse restaurant menus online before your visit to make an informed decision.
Please do not hesitate to ask questions. If you have any questions about the menu, ask the waiter. They should help you choose healthy options that you enjoy. Making healthy choices at a restaurant can be difficult, but it's definitely possible. By following these tips, you can make healthy choices that will help you reach your weight loss goals.

Chapter 3: Getting active

1/ How much exercise do you need

The Centers for Disease Control and Prevention (CDC) recommends that adults do at least
150 minutes of moderate-intensity aerobic activity or 75 minutes of vigorous-intensity aerobic
activity each week.
The American College of Sports Medicine (ACSM) recommends at least 30 minutes of
moderate-intensity aerobic activity for adults most days of the week.
The amount of exercise you need depends on your age, fitness level, and health goals.
It is also important to do strength training at least twice a week.
Strength training helps build muscle and burn calories. Here are some examples of moderate-
intensity aerobic exercise.

- brisk walking
- cycle
- dance
- swimming
- water aerobics
- row
- jumping jack
- sprint
- HIIT (High Intensity Interval Training)
- Tennis, basketball, football …

If you are new to the sport, start slowly and gradually increase your weekly training time.
Also, you should consult your doctor before starting any new exercise program.

Here are some additional tips for getting active.

Find an activity that you enjoy. That way, you're more likely to keep doing it.
Set realistic goals. Don't try to do too many things too quickly. Start with small goals and
gradually increase your weekly training time.

Find a training partner. If you have someone to train with, keep yourself motivated.
Make exercise part of your routine. Make time to exercise during the day and stick to it.
Don't be afraid to take breaks. If you need a break, take a break. Resume exercise as soon as
possible.

Staying active is key to losing weight and improving your overall health. By following these
tips, you can make exercise a part of your life and reach your weight loss goals.

2/What types of exercise are best for weight loss

- **Aerobic**: Aerobic exercise is any type of exercise that gets your heart rate up and your breathing rough. Examples of aerobic exercise include brisk walking, running, swimming, cycling, and dancing. Aerobic exercise burns calories and is great for weight loss.
- **strength training**: Strength training is any type of exercise that helps build muscle. Examples of strength training include lifting weights, using resistance bands, and bodyweight exercises such as push-ups and squats. Strength training is important for weight loss because it helps you burn more calories at rest.
- **Interval training**: Interval training is a type of training that alternates between short bursts of high-intensity training and short breaks. Interval training is a great way to burn calories and improve fitness.
- **HIIT** : High-intensity interval training is a type of very high-intensity interval training. HIIT workouts are usually short, lasting only 10-30 minutes. However, it is very effective at burning calories and improving fitness.

It is important to choose an exercise that is enjoyable and sustainable. If you don't like exercise, you are less likely to exercise regularly. Also, you should consult your doctor before starting any new exercise program.

<u>Here are some additional tips for choosing the right kind of weight loss workout.</u>

Consider your fitness level. If you are new to sports, start with low-intensity cardio. As you get stronger, gradually increase the intensity of your exercise.
Find an activity that you enjoy. That way, you're more likely to keep doing it.
Add variety to your training. This will help you avoid boredom and plateaus.
Listen to your body. Take a break if you feel pain.
The best exercise for weight loss is exercise that is enjoyable and sustainable. By following these tips, you can find the type of exercise that works for you and reach your weight loss goals.

3/How to stay motivated

Set clear goals for yourself. What do you want to achieve? Once you know what you need, you can break it down into smaller, more manageable steps. By doing so, it will become less difficult and more achievable.
Visualize your success. How do you feel when you reach your goal? What can you achieve? Imagining your own success helps you stay motivated in difficult situations.
Reward yourself for your achievements. Reward yourself with small rewards when you reach a milestone. That way, you can stay on track and stay motivated to keep going.
Find a support system. Talk to your friends, family and colleagues about your goals. They will offer encouragement and support when needed.
Get a break. Don't try to do it all at once. Take breaks throughout the day to relax and recharge your energy. This will help you stay focused and motivated.
Celebrate your progress. Don't just focus on the end goal. Celebrate your progress along the way. This will help you stay motivated and stay on track.
Here are some additional tips to help you stay motivated.

find a mentor. Find someone who has already achieved what you want to achieve. They can provide guidance and support. Read motivational books and articles. This will help you stay inspired and motivated.

Listen to music that motivates you. This will help you stay healthy and ready for anything.

Watch motivational videos. This is a great way to get inspired and motivated.

Meditate or practice mindfulness. This will help you clear your head and focus on your goals.

take care. Make sure you get enough sleep, eat healthy, and exercise regularly. It will help you feel better and keep you motivated.

Remember, motivation is not constant. There are high tides and high tides. Sometimes you get motivated, sometimes you don't. The most important thing is to never give up. Keep taking steps toward your goals, even if you feel discouraged. You will eventually reach your goal.

Chapter 4: Overcoming common challenges

1/How to deal with cravings

Food cravings are a normal part of life, but they can be especially difficult when trying to change a healthy diet. Here are some tips on how to deal with your appetite.

Identify your triggers. What makes you want to eat unhealthy foods? Knowing what causes them can help you avoid them or find healthy ways to deal with them.
Eat regular meals and snacks. This helps keep you feeling full and prevents excessive hunger that can lead to hunger.
Choose healthy foods that you enjoy. If you don't enjoy what you eat, you're more likely to lose your appetite. Have healthy snacks and meals on hand that you actually look forward to eating.
drink lots of water. Thirst is sometimes confused with hunger. So make sure you drink enough water throughout the day.
Get enough sleep When you don't get enough sleep, your body produces more of the stress hormone cortisol, which can trigger your appetite.
Find healthy ways to deal with stress. When you're stressed, it's important to find healthy ways to deal with it. Exercise, relaxation techniques, and spending time with loved ones can help reduce stress and reduce cravings for unhealthy foods.
Don't blame yourself for giving in to desire. Everyone gives in to their own desires from time to time. The important thing is to keep trying and not give up.
Here are some additional tips to help control your appetite.

distract yourself. If you feel an appetite, try to distract yourself with something else. Go for a walk, read a book, or do any other activity you enjoy.
If you're having trouble coping with your appetite to talk to someone, talk to someone you trust. They can offer support and encouragement. Join our support group. There are many groups that support people trying to change their diet to become healthier. Joining a support group helps you stay motivated and learn from others who feel the same way.
Remember that desires are temporary. If you just leave it alone, it will come back someday. Don't give up and keep trying.

2/How to deal with plateaus

A weight loss plateau is a normal part of the weight loss process. It can be frustrating, but there are things you can do to overcome it.

Here are some tips for dealing with the weight loss plateau.
Rethink your goals. Are you still on the right track to reach your goals? If not, you may need to adjust your goals and approach. Please review your eating habits. Are you still eating healthy and sticking to your calorie budget? If not, you may need to make some changes.
Step up your training. Adding more exercise to your routine will help you burn more calories and break plateaus. Rest Sometimes you just need a break from your weight loss journey. Take a few days off diet and exercise and come back refreshed.
be patient. The weight loss plateau is frustrating, but it's temporary. If you keep at it, you'll eventually break through.
Here are some additional tips to help you overcome the weight loss plateau.

Change your diet. If you eat three large meals a day, try smaller, more frequent meals. This helps keep your metabolism up.

Try intermittent fasting. Intermittent fasting is a popular weight loss method that alternates between eating and fasting periods. This will help you burn more fat and break plateaus.

Add strength training to your routine. Strength training can help build muscle, boost your metabolism, and increase your resting calorie burn.

get enough sleep Lack of sleep causes your body to produce more of the stress hormone cortisol, which can lead to weight gain.

stress management. Stress can also lead to weight gain. Find healthy ways to deal with stress, such as exercise, yoga, and meditation.

Note that the weight loss plateau is temporary. If you keep at it, you'll eventually break through.

3/How to deal with setbacks

Setbacks are inevitable in any weight loss journey. You may be discouraged, but that doesn't mean you have to give up.

Here are some tips on how to deal with setbacks:

Don't blame yourself. Everyone has setbacks. Most importantly, don't judge yourself. Pick yourself up and move on.

Determine the cause of the kickback. What caused it to go off track? Once you know the cause, you can start making changes to avoid future problems.

Don't give up on your goals. You don't have to give up on your goals just because you've experienced setbacks. Keep striving towards them and you will eventually reach them.

Notice the progress we've made so far. It's easy to focus on setbacks, but it's also important to focus on the progress you've made. Remember how far you've come and don't let setbacks slow you down. Get back on track as soon as possible. Try not to prolong the recoil. Get back on track as soon as possible so you can reach your goals.

Here are some additional tips to help you deal with setbacks.

Talk to someone If you find it difficult to deal with a setback, talk to someone you trust. They can offer support and encouragement.

Join our support group. There are many support groups for people who want to lose weight. Joining a support group helps you stay motivated and learn from others who feel the same way.

Rest. Sometimes you just need a break from your weight loss journey. Take a few days off diet and exercise and come back refreshed.

Remember that setbacks are temporary. If you keep at it, you will eventually reach your goal.

Chapter 5: Maintaining your weight loss

1/How to keep the weight off

<u>Here are some tips for maintaining your weight after losing it.</u>

Make a healthy change in your lifestyle. This means making changes that are sustainable over the long term. This includes eating healthy, exercising regularly, and getting enough sleep. Don't go back to old habits. This is the most important tip. If you go back to your old lifestyle, you may gain weight again. Therefore, it's important to find ways to maintain a healthy lifestyle.
be patient. Maintaining weight loss takes time. Don't expect to see results overnight. If you keep at it, you will eventually reach your goal.
Please do not give up. There will be times when you want to give up. However, it is important not to give up. Just keep going and eventually you will reach your goal. Here are some additional tips to help you maintain your weight loss.

Set realistic goals. Don't try to lose weight too quickly. This is a recipe for failure. Set realistic goals that are achievable and sustainable.
Track your progress. This will help you stay motivated and stay on track. There are many ways to track your progress, such as using a food diary or fitness tracker.
Find a support system. Having someone to support you makes a big difference. This may include friends, family, or weight loss groups. Don't be afraid to ask for help. If you're having trouble maintaining your weight loss, don't be afraid to seek help from your doctor, nutritionist, or therapist.
Remember that maintaining weight loss is a journey. There will be ups and downs, but if you persevere, you will definitely reach your goals.

2/How to prevent yo-yo dieting

The yo-yo diet causes weight loss and weight gain, which can be detrimental to your health. Here are some tips to prevent yo-yo dieting.

Change your lifestyle gradually. Don't try to change too quickly. This is a recipe for failure. Make incremental changes that are sustainable over time. Focus on healthy changes, not just weight loss. That means eating healthy, exercising regularly, and getting enough sleep. If you focus on making healthy changes, the weight will come off naturally.
Don't over-restrict your calorie intake. If you restrict your calorie intake too much, you are more likely to restrict your calorie intake and gain weight back. Aim to lose 1-2 pounds per week.
Don't blame yourself for setbacks. Everyone has setbacks. If you encounter setbacks, don't worry. Get back on track and keep going. Find a support system. Having someone to support you makes a big difference. This may include friends, family, or weight loss groups.
Don't be afraid to ask for help. If you're having trouble avoiding the yo-yo diet, don't be afraid to ask your doctor, dietitian, or therapist for help. Remember, the yo-yo diet is a tough cycle to break. But if you make gradual lifestyle changes and focus on healthy changes, you can break the cycle and reach your weight loss goals.

<u>Here are some additional tips to help prevent yo-yo dieting.</u>

Find healthy ways to deal with stress. Stress can lead to unhealthy eating habits, so it's important to find healthy ways to manage stress. Exercise, yoga, and meditation may help. Learn to listen to your body. Watch out for hunger signs and eat when you're hungry. don't try to starve.

Don't label food as "good" or "bad." All foods can be incorporated into a healthy diet. Focus on eating healthy foods in moderation. Take time for yourself. It's important to take care of yourself, both physically and mentally. Make time for activities that you enjoy and relax. Remember, the yo-yo diet is a tough cycle to break. But if you make gradual lifestyle changes and focus on healthy changes, you can break the cycle and reach your weight loss goals.

Conclusion

Set realistic goals. Don't try to lose weight too quickly. This is a recipe for failure. Set realistic goals that are achievable and sustainable.
Make a healthy change in your lifestyle. This means making changes that are sustainable over the long term. This includes eating healthy, exercising regularly, and getting enough sleep.
Don't go back to old habits. This is the most important tip. If you go back to your old lifestyle, you may end up gaining weight again. Therefore, it's important to find ways to maintain a healthy lifestyle.
be patient. Losing and maintaining weight takes time. Don't expect to see results overnight. If you keep at it, you will eventually reach your goal. Please do not give up. There will be times when you want to give up. However, it is important not to give up. Just keep going and you will eventually reach your goal.